PAUL ANDREW MILLER

Embracing the Outdoors

The Profound Benefits of Spending Time in Nature

This book was professionally typeset on Reedsy.
Find out more at reedsy.com

In every walk with nature, one receives far
more than he seeks.

John Muir

Contents

1

Embracing the Outdoors

Introduction

Nature has a profound way of touching our lives, often in ways we don't fully realize until we immerse ourselves in its beauty. Consider the story of John Muir, the renowned naturalist who found solace and inspiration in the wilderness. His writings describe how his time in nature not only invigorated his body but also his mind and spirit. Such stories are not unique to Muir; they echo through the lives of countless individuals who have discovered the transformative power of the natural world.

In our fast-paced, technology-driven society, the importance of reconnecting with nature cannot be overstated. Nature offers a sanctuary from the stresses of modern life, providing numerous benefits that span physical health, mental well-being, social connections, environmental awareness, and personal growth. This book aims to delve into these multifaceted benefits, offering insights into why spending time outdoors is vital for our overall health and happiness.

We will explore how outdoor activities can enhance cardiovascular health, boost the immune system, improve sleep quality, and aid in weight management. We'll also examine mental health benefits, including stress reduction, improved mood, enhanced cognitive function, and the alleviation of anxiety and depression. The special role exposure to sunlight plays in both these areas will also be addressed. Social advantages, such as strengthening relationships and building communities, will be considered, along with the role of nature in fostering environmental stewardship and education.

Furthermore, we'll reflect on the spiritual and personal growth that can come from spending time in nature, ranging from fostering a connection to something greater than ourselves to inspiring creativity and mindfulness. Practical tips for integrating nature into daily life will be provided, encouraging readers to incorporate these benefits into their routines.

Understanding these positive effects is crucial in today's world, where many people are increasingly disconnected from nature, spending a great deal of their time indoors. By the end of this book, readers will be inspired to embrace the outdoors, reaping the myriad benefits it has to offer.

2

Physical Health Benefits

Improved Cardiovascular Health

Outdoor activities such as hiking, cycling, running, and especially just walking are excellent ways to improve cardiovascular health. Engaging in these activities regularly can lead to lower blood pressure, improved cholesterol levels, and a reduced risk of heart disease. Research has shown that even moderate exercise in a natural setting can significantly boost heart health. In fact, studies have found that people who simply live near green spaces have lower rates of cardiovascular disease (Keith et al., 2024).

The fresh air and varied terrain encountered during outdoor activities provide a more dynamic workout compared to indoor exercises. This variability helps improve cardiovascular endurance and strength. Additionally, the natural beauty of outdoor settings can make exercise feel less like a chore and more like an enjoyable activity, encouraging people to stay active longer. Most people would agree that a 20-minute walk in nature is more appealing than 20 minutes on a treadmill at the gym.

Enhanced Immune Function

Exposure to fresh air and sunlight plays a crucial role in boosting the immune system. Sunlight is a natural source of vitamin D, which is essential for maintaining a healthy immune response. Regular exposure to natural environments can enhance immune function, making the body more resilient against infections and diseases. Some believe a shadow has been cast on the issue of exposure to UV radiation by the risks associated with sunburn. However, the National Institutes of Health recommend sun exposure daily for 5 to 30 minutes most days a week without sunscreen, as even SPF 8 or less may block the body's ability to absorb the UVB rays that stimulate effective vitamin D3 production (Srivastava, 2021b).

Activities like gardening, hiking, and simply spending time in green spaces, especially forests, have been shown to increase the activity of natural killer cells, a type of white blood cell that plays a critical role in the body's defense against viruses and tumors (Very Big Brain, 2024). This effect is linked especially with the practice of forest bathing, known in Japan as *shinrin-yoku*, which is described as "...the conscious and contemplative practice of being immersed in the sights, sounds and smells of the forest" (Global Wellness Institute, 2022b). Studies conducted there on the benefits of forest bathing demonstrate that spending time in forests can indeed enhance immune function by increasing both the number of these cells and their activity. This effect was found to last for more than seven days. Reduced stress was also apparent as a significant decrease in the levels of cortisol and adrenaline was also found.

Better Sleep Quality

Natural light is a key regulator of our circadian rhythms, the body's internal clock that governs sleep-wake cycles. Exposure to natural light during the day helps maintain a healthy circadian rhythm, leading to better sleep quality at night. Studies have shown that people who spend more time outdoors tend to fall asleep faster and enjoy deeper, more restful sleep.

As many as 70% of those over the age of 65 report chronic sleep problems. Research indicates that a contributing factor could be light deficiency, which is exacerbated through aging, as this reduces the ability of the eyes to benefit from the stimulation of sunlight, which will be explored in more depth below.

The calming effects of nature also contribute to improved sleep. Spending time in natural settings reduces stress and anxiety, creating a more relaxed state conducive to sleep. Anecdotal evidence shows that individuals who spend weekends camping or hiking often report significantly better sleep during and after their outdoor experiences.

Some readers may remember their mothers telling them to go outdoors to get some fresh air so they would be able to sleep better. Scientific research has often substantiated such items of folk wisdom. Throughout Europe, many people routinely seek to enhance their sleep quality by leaving a window open in the bedroom overnight, essentially inviting nature indoors to work its magic with them while sleeping.

Weight Management and Obesity Prevention

Outdoor activities offer a fun and engaging way to stay physically active, which is essential for weight management and obesity prevention. Unlike indoor exercises, outdoor activities provide a constantly changing environment that keeps the mind engaged and the body challenged.

Whether it's hiking up a mountain, cycling along a forest trail, or playing a game of soccer in the park, these activities help burn calories and build muscle. This contributes to the development of what we could call a positive feedback loop. Muscles burn more calories than fat, no matter whether we are active or at rest, which means the body's basal metabolic rate increases as we put on more muscle. Consequently, we enjoy the double benefit of both burning calories while exercising and, due to increased muscle mass, automatically burning more calories while the body merely performs its basic life-sustaining functions, whether sitting on the couch, resting or even sleeping.

Research has shown that people who engage in regular outdoor exercise are more likely to maintain a healthy weight compared to those who primarily exercise indoors. The combination of physical exertion, fresh air, and the enjoyment of being in nature makes outdoor activities an effective and sustainable way to help manage weight.

The Importance of Sunlight

Sunlight deserves special mention here because of its importance for both physical and mental health. The retina of the human eye contains photosensitive cells connected directly to the brain—completely apart from the function of vision. Sunlight, especially the short-wavelength spectrum of blue light just beyond the visible range, stimulates these cells positively. This facilitates the proper function of the pineal gland, the pituitary gland, and the hypothalamus in the brain, meaning that sunlight is essential for brain health directly as well as for physiological health in a broader sense.

The body's internal, or biological, clock referred to earlier is controlled by the hypothalamus. This encompasses far more than just the body's sleep patterns, however. Most cells in the body operate cyclically, meaning that disruptions in their cycles due to a lack of light stimulation can potentially have a detrimental effect on nearly any area of the body. The consequences can include physiological and psychological aspects and even an increase in the risk of disease because of the central role the hypothalamus plays in regulating the combined actions of the hormonal and nervous systems.

The pineal gland produces melatonin, which, apart from its more well-known role in sleep/wake cycle regulation, also helps protect our skin and is a powerful antioxidant that works throughout the body. Not only is it a key for sleep quality, but also for the function of our intestines, and it can help prevent depression.

If you are one of those people who don't quite feel alive until after that first cup of coffee in the morning, here is a tip that can help you wake up faster so you can enjoy your coffee for more than its effect. The transition from sleep to wakefulness requires the function of the adrenal glands, which are influenced by the pituitary and hypothalamus in the brain. As those photosensitive cells in our eyes stimulate the brain, we can kick-start the entire process of coming alive after sleep by taking a peek outside at the first sunlight of dawn—especially without a window pane. We're not talking about foolishly staring into the sun, but exposing our eyes to the natural light of the outdoors. Try it. You just might find it habit-forming!

3

Mental Health Benefits

Stress Reduction

Nature has a remarkable ability to reduce stress. The sights, sounds, and smells of natural environments trigger a relaxation response in the body, lowering cortisol levels and reducing overall stress. The affinity to nature expressed by these phenomena is known as biophilia, a concept that suggests humans have an innate connection to nature that promotes well–being.

Personal stories and expert opinions abound, illustrating how time spent in nature can melt away the stresses of modern life. For example, individuals who participate in wilderness therapy programs often report significant reductions in stress and improvements in mental health. These programs utilize the therapeutic benefits of nature to help people cope with anxiety, depression, and other mental health issues.

One nationwide study of over 900,000 people compared the long-term mental health of adolescents and adults based on the amount of green space available to them as children. Those who grew up with the least green space had an up to 55% greater risk of developing a psychiatric disorder than those who grew up with the most green space. This was the result after making adjustments for other risk factors, such as urbanization, socioeconomic factors, family history of mental illness, and parental age (Engemann et al., 2019).

Improved Mood and Happiness

Spending time outdoors has been shown to improve mood and increase happiness. The connection between time in nature and elevated serotonin levels is well-documented. Serotonin is a neurotransmitter that contributes to feelings of well-being and happiness. Engaging in outdoor activities, whether a leisurely walk in the park or an adventurous hike, can boost serotonin levels and enhance overall mood.

Research findings consistently support the mood-boosting effects of nature. A study published in the journal Environmental Science & Technology found that individuals who spent time in a natural setting experienced significant improvements in mood and self-esteem within just five minutes (Barton & Pretty, 2010). This effect was even more pronounced in people who engaged in physical activity while outdoors.

My own walks in the forest begin with about ten minutes of striding through an urban residential area. While this is good for my body, my soul and spirit experience a significant lift only once I enter the forest. The late afternoon sunlight slanting through the branches with their needles in "my" coniferous woods combined with the aromatic pungency of the sun-warmed sap are a soothing balm that takes effect quickly as it surrounds me.

Enhanced Cognitive Function

Outdoor activities have been shown to enhance cognitive function, including improved focus, creativity, and problem-solving skills. The natural environment provides a break from the constant stimuli of urban life, allowing the brain to rest and rejuvenate. This phenomenon, known as attention restoration theory, suggests that exposure to nature helps replenish cognitive resources, improving mental clarity and focus.

Examples from educational and professional settings demonstrate the cognitive benefits of outdoor activities. Schools that incorporate outdoor learning and play into their curriculum often report better academic performance and improved behavior among students. Similarly, professionals who take breaks in natural settings or participate in outdoor team-building activities often experience increased productivity and creativity.

Reduction in Anxiety and Depression

Nature serves as a complementary therapy for anxiety and depression. The calming effects of natural environments, combined with physical activity and social interaction, create a powerful antidote to these mental health challenges. Studies have shown that people who spend time in nature experience lower levels of anxiety and depression compared to those who spend most of their time indoors.

Relevant psychological studies and real-life examples highlight the therapeutic benefits of nature. For instance, a study published in the journal Landscape and Urban Planning found that individuals who walked in a natural setting for 90 minutes reported lower levels of rumination, a key factor in depression, compared to those who walked in an urban environment (*The Benefits of Nature Experience: Improved Affect and Cognition*, 2015b). Nature's ability to soothe the mind and spirit makes it an effective tool in the treatment and prevention of mental health issues. In fact, hiking is now being used as a counseling approach that seeks to combine the benefits of nature with conventional psychotherapy for a synergistic effect.

4

Social Benefits

Strengthening Relationships

Outdoor activities provide an excellent opportunity to bond with family and friends. Shared experiences in nature create lasting memories and strengthen relationships. Especially active endeavors, such as hiking and walking, provide the backdrop of regular bodily motion as each step is taken, which leaves the mind and spirit free for engagement, not only with oneself, but also with others. Whether it's a hike in the woods, a family camping trip, biking with friends, or a day at the beach, these activities all foster connection and communication.

Examples of group activities and their social benefits abound. Families who regularly engage in outdoor activities often report stronger bonds and improved communication. Friendships are also strengthened through shared adventures and challenges in nature, creating a sense of camaraderie and mutual support. This even takes place between strangers as an unexpected encounter with a special or rare event in a natural setting can quickly overcome social distance. While traveling through Rocky Mountain National Park, I quickly discovered that a traffic jam was often the first indication of a wildlife sighting. Elk or moose grazing in a meadow beside the road draw people out of their cars and into conversation with others they have never met before. While such interactions are brief and spontaneous, they serve as a reminder of the positive effect intentional time spent in nature with friends and family can have.

Building Community

Nature has the power to bring people together and build communities. Community gardens, parks, and outdoor events provide spaces for people to connect and engage with one another. Sharing the outdoors with others eliminates the host–guest interface that often accompanies visits in other people's homes or personal spaces. This fosters social connections and often creates a more relaxed sense of belonging. We saw in Chapter 2 that we are calmer in nature, but we are also often kinder, too.

A story is told of a biologist in Eastern Siberia who was studying the area's wildlife. He expected to find that the strongest animals survived the best, in line with the "survival of the fittest" theory prevalent in his day in the nineteenth century. Instead, he discovered that the animals who fared best in the challenging environment of Siberia were the ones that cooperated with other species (Creating Community Through Nature, 2022a). Studies of successful community initiatives that involve nature among humans illustrate the same social benefits found in the wild. For instance, urban gardening projects not only provide fresh produce but also create a sense of community among participants. Similarly, outdoor festivals and events draw people together, promoting social interaction and cultural exchange.

Enhancing Social Skills in Children

Nature plays a crucial role in the social development of children. Outdoor play and exploration provide opportunities for children to interact with their peers, develop social skills, and build friendships. Research has shown that children who spend more time outdoors are more likely to exhibit positive social behaviors and have better social skills. One study with eighty students from an urban Canadian elementary school demonstrated that more positive social effects resulted from a field trip to a nature school than a visit to an aviation and space museum (Dopko et al., 2019).

Other studies on play and social interaction in natural settings also highlight the benefits of outdoor activities for children's social development. For example, children who participate in nature-based education programs often demonstrate improved teamwork, communication, and problem-solving skills. The unstructured, imaginative play that occurs in natural environments fosters creativity and social competence.

5

Environmental Awareness and Stewardship

Increased Environmental Consciousness

Spending time in nature fosters a sense of responsibility towards the environment. When people connect with nature, they develop a deeper appreciation not only for its beauty, but also for its complexity. This connection often translates into a greater commitment to environmental conservation and sustainability.

Examples of individuals and groups who became environmental advocates after spending time in nature are numerous. For instance, many environmentalists credit their passion for conservation to childhood experiences in nature. That middle age of childhood between the ages of about five and eleven seems to be an especially formative time. When a love for nature is fostered, especially under the guidance of a trusted adult, knowledge will surely follow. These experiences often inspire lifelong commitments to engaging with and protecting the environment.

Promoting Conservation Efforts

Outdoor experiences play a significant role in supporting conservation initiatives. People who spend time in nature are more likely to participate in conservation efforts and advocate for environmental protection. This involvement can range from volunteering for local clean-up projects to supporting national and international conservation organizations.

Case studies of conservation projects inspired by nature experiences highlight the impact of outdoor activities on environmental stewardship. For example, many successful conservation projects were initiated by individuals who were moved by their experiences in nature to take action. These projects often involve community participation and education, further promoting environmental awareness.

Educational Benefits

Outdoor education programs have a profound impact on environmental awareness. These programs teach participants about the natural world and the importance of conservation. Yet it is often through hands-on learning experiences that participants gain a deeper understanding of ecological principles and develop a sense of stewardship.

Testimonials from educators and students involved in outdoor education programs underscore the educational benefits of nature. Students who participate in these programs often report increased knowledge and appreciation of the environment. Educators also note improvements in student engagement and academic performance, as well as a greater sense of responsibility towards the environment.

6

Spiritual and Personal Growth

Connection to Something Greater

Nature inspires a sense of spirituality and connectedness. Many people find that spending time in nature helps them feel connected to something greater than themselves. This connection can take many forms, from a sense of awe and wonder at the beauty of the natural world to a feeling of spiritual transcendence or encounter with a higher power.

Quotes and stories from different cultural and spiritual backgrounds highlight the spiritual benefits of nature. For example, many indigenous cultures have deep spiritual connections to the land and view nature as sacred. Similarly, individuals from various religious and spiritual traditions often describe profound spiritual experiences in natural settings. For instance, John Muir's dedication to nature led him to believe that "God's love is manifest in the landscape as in a face" (*The Cruise of the Corwin* by John Muir, n.d.).

Personal Reflection and Mindfulness

Nature provides an ideal setting for personal reflection and mindfulness. The tranquility and beauty of natural environments create a space for introspection and self-discovery. Practices such as forest bathing or mindful forest walking help individuals connect with their inner selves and find clarity and peace. Spending time mindfully in a beautiful location can help cement its memory within you, creating a place to which you can return mentally even when separated from the physical location by thousands of miles. When surrounded by challenging circumstances, or even simply in the midst of everyday events, this can be a source from which to draw renewed focus and strength and experience peace and clarity.

The benefits of solitude in nature for personal reflection are well-documented. Many people find that spending time alone in nature helps them gain perspective on their lives and make important decisions. The practice of mindfulness in nature, whether through meditation or simply being present in the moment, enhances mental clarity and emotional well-being.

It is reported that people have about 300 "self-talk" thoughts a minute. These usually revolve about oneself, fostering self-absorption, not reflection. The sensory activities entailed in spending time in nature help break through our self-preoccupation, inviting us to engage with the world outside. By becoming aware, worry and stress melt away and we are able to rediscover and focus on positive truths (Creating Community Through Nature, 2022a).

In my own experience, rock climbing has proven to be the fastest route for me to shed the cares and concerns that can preoccupy the mind and soul. The fully absorbing mental and physical interaction with the rock contours immediately before my face drain all else away as I use handholds and footholds to move up the pitch. This total engagement at once both narrows my focus to the immediacy of accomplishing the next move and enhances the exhilarating sense of freedom afforded by the experience of overcoming gravity to ascend a vertical wall of rock as I am captivated by the moment.

Inspiration and Creativity

Nature is a powerful source of inspiration and creativity. Many artists, writers, and thinkers draw inspiration from the natural world. The beauty and complexity of nature spark creativity and innovative thinking, leading to the creation of art, literature, and scientific discoveries.

Examples of individuals inspired by nature to create remarkable works abound. For instance, the poet William Wordsworth wrote many of his famous works while walking in the Lake District. Henry David Thoreau lived beside Walden Pond for two years. He spent hours walking through and interacting with the nature that surrounded him. His attempt to live by the rhythms of the natural world and his detailed observations of it are recorded in what is perhaps his most well-known work, the book Walden (Whitworth, 2023b). In their quest for powered human flight, the Wright brothers also found inspiration in nature. Orville is reported to have meditated on the wing warping of birds in flight. He identified this focus on nature's example as being a pivotal factor in their success. This principle of biomimicry continues to be important as man learns from nature, seeking to emulate it to solve complex human problems (Wikipedia contributors, 2024d). Nature's ability to inspire creativity is a testament to its profound impact on the human spirit.

$$7$$

Practical Tips for Integrating Nature into Daily Life

Finding Nature Nearby

Discovering local parks, trails, and natural spots is easier than ever, thanks to modern technology. There are numerous resources and apps available that help people locate nearby nature areas. Websites and apps like AllTrails and Google Maps can guide you to local parks and hiking trails. Or simply do an Internet search for possibilities near you.

Exploring nature doesn't always require a trip to a remote wilderness. Many urban areas have hidden pockets of green space that provide a quick and accessible escape from the hustle and bustle of city life. Look for community gardens, urban parks, and nature reserves in your area.

Developing an awareness of even brief encounters with pockets of nature when outdoors in an urban context can have a positive effect. For instance, while I cycle home from the city center along an urban bike route, one of these encounters with nature takes place as the bike path joins the course of a babbling stream for a quarter of a mile. The gentle sound of the water flowing over stones is immediately soothing. Another is with an evergreen hedge that exudes a pleasant piney smell that I enjoy for the ten seconds it takes me to pass by. As fleeting as such encounters may be, practicing mindfulness and looking for the presence of nature purposefully is a worthwhile endeavor. As we do so, we may find ourselves surprised at the amount of nature we discover.

Incorporating Outdoor Activities

Making time for outdoor activities in a busy schedule can be challenging, but it's possible with a bit of planning. Start by setting aside specific times each week for outdoor activities, such as weekend hikes or evening walks. Incorporate nature into your daily routine by walking or cycling to work. Many urban areas have made great strides in promoting cycling for both commuting and recreational purposes, but commuting by bike gives you two benefits for the price of one: fitness and encounters with nature—even three if we count the advantages that accrue to the environment.

Taking breaks in nearby parks, or having lunch outdoors are also ways to make room for nature. When I worked in a factory with no windows, I went outdoors for nearly every break, but at least for lunchtime. Walking out into the sunshine, closing my eyes and feeling the warming radiation of the sun's presence offered a welcome respite, melting away workday tensions—even if for only 5 minutes.

Family-friendly activities like picnics, nature walks, and outdoor sports are excellent ways to spend quality time together while enjoying the benefits of nature. For individuals, activities like bird watching, photography, or simply reading a book in a park can provide a refreshing break enhanced by the presence of nature.

Creating a Nature-Friendly Environment at Home

Bringing elements of nature into your home can create a calming and rejuvenating atmosphere. Indoor plants are a simple and effective way to incorporate nature into your living space. They not only enhance the aesthetic appeal of your home but also improve air quality. While they may not scrub the air as well as modern air purifiers, they are certainly quieter and more attractive. Other benefits have been shown to include improving mood, reducing stress levels, boosting productivity and increasing our ability to concentrate.

Maximize natural light by keeping windows unobstructed and using light, airy curtains. Sunlight has a much broader light spectrum than traditional artificial lighting and this is associated with positive physical and psychological effects. Natural light governs the production of melatonin and serotonin in the body. In the absence of light, the body produces melatonin, which is important in regulating our sleep-wake cycle, the circadian rhythm. Serotonin, on the other hand, is a hormone that helps boost mood and its production is stimulated by natural light. Modern lifestyles that entail spending a great deal of time indoors with artificial lighting can impair these natural regulators.

Also consider creating an outdoor living space, such as a balcony garden or a patio with comfortable seating, where you can relax and enjoy the light and fresh air. There is no need to bake in the sun. An awning or umbrella can provide pleasant shade while the natural light with its positive effects still reaches us. This becomes evident when we consider how many people still wear sunglasses even when seated under a sun umbrella.

Humans seem to be so tuned in to nature that even watching nature documentaries or videos can have a positive effect on our well-being. A study published in the Journal of Environmental Psychology found many of the emotional well-being effects that result from interacting with real nature mentioned earlier were also evident when study participants viewed nature on TV. A digital dose of virtual nature was found to reduce negative feelings such as sadness or boredom. Perhaps surprisingly, computer-generated virtual reality interaction with nature provided a significantly greater improvement in the positive effects than did merely watching TV (Yeo et al., 2020).

Planning Nature Trips and Adventures

Planning nature trips and adventures can be an exciting way to explore new places and enjoy the great outdoors. Whether it's a weekend camping trip, a hiking excursion, or a vacation to a national park, careful planning ensures a safe and enjoyable experience.

When planning a nature trip, research the destination to understand what to expect in terms of terrain, weather, and available facilities. Pack appropriate gear and supplies, and prioritize safety by informing someone of your plans and checking in at appropriate intervals, especially when venturing out into the wild. Consider joining guided tours or outdoor groups if you're new to nature excursions, as they can provide valuable knowledge and support.

8

Conclusion

Throughout this book, we've explored the myriad benefits of spending time in nature. From improved physical health to enhanced mental well-being, from strengthened social connections to increased environmental awareness, nature offers countless advantages that enrich our lives. We've seen how nature can reduce stress, boost mood, and inspire creativity, while also fostering a sense of community and stewardship.

The transformative power of nature is evident in the stories and studies we've discussed. Nature's ability to heal, inspire, and connect us is unparalleled. Humankind's connectedness to nature, reflected in the concept of biophilia, is a medium that facilitates the emergence of these, sometimes unexpected and sometimes awe-inspiring, effects. In a world where many of us are increasingly disconnected from the natural world and each other, it's more important than ever to recognize and embrace the benefits of spending time outdoors.

I encourage you to take steps toward integrating nature into your daily life. Whether it's a simple walk in the park, a weekend camping trip, or creating a green space at home, make a conscious effort to connect with nature. Engage all of your senses to mindfully interact with the natural environment that surrounds you. Even in spaces where nature seems to struggle to assert itself, it can still be found and appreciated. The benefits you'll experience—physically, mentally, and spiritually—will be well worth the effort.

As John Muir once said, "In every walk with nature, one receives far more than he seeks (Wood, n.d.)." I initially overlooked Muir's choice of preposition, with. Yet upon reflection, I find it strikingly appropriate. In our interactions with other humans, we sometimes find ourselves talking at them instead of with them. The same danger exists when engaging nature in the great outdoors. An attitude of mindfulness and attentiveness to all that nature not only has to offer, but is, is essential—and enriching. Let this quote inspire you to step outside, embrace the outdoors, and discover the profound benefits that nature abundantly provides.

If you found this book helpful, I'd be very appreciative if you would leave a favorable review for the book on Amazon!

9

References and Further Reading

Books and Articles

"The Nature Fix: Why Nature Makes Us Happier, Healthier, and More Creative" by Florence Williams

"Last Child in the Woods: Saving Our Children from Nature-Deficit Disorder" by Richard Louv

"Your Brain on Nature: The Science of Nature's Influence on Your Health, Happiness and Vitality" by Eva M. Selhub and Alan C. Logan

Organizations

Sierra Club (*https://www.sierraclub.org/*)

National Park Foundation (*https://www.nationalparks.org/*)

The Nature Conservancy (*https://www.nature.org/*)

AllTrails (*https://www.alltrails.com/*)

1. Nature Sacred (*https://naturesacred.org/*)
2. Leave No Trace Center for Outdoor Ethics (*https://lnt.org/*)

Resources

Keith, R. J., Hart, J. L., & Bhatnagar, A. (2024). Greenspaces and cardiovascular health. *Circulation Research, 134*(9), 1179–1196. *https://doi.org/10.1161/circresaha.124.323583*

Srivastava, S. B. (2021). Vitamin D: Do we need more than sunshine? *American Journal of Lifestyle Medicine,* 155982762110056. *https://doi.org/10.1177/15598276211005689*
    https://www.ncbi.nlm.nih.gov/pmc/articles/PMC8299926/#:~:text=Vitamin%20D%20From%20the%20Sun&text=It%20is%20optimal%20to%20have,to%20effectively%20make%20vitamin%20D

Very Big Brain. (2024, April 1). *Biophilia: How love of life and nature impact brain function.* Very Big Brain. *https://verybigbrain.com/outside-influences/biophilia-how-love-of-life-and-nature-impact-brain-function/*

Global Wellness Institute. (2022, September 15). *Forest Bathing - Global Wellness Institute.* *https://globalwellnessinstitute.org/wellnessevidence/forest-bathing/#:~:text=A%20small%202017%20Nippon%20Medical,cancer%20proteins%2C%20while%20significantly%20decreasing*

Maffetone, P. (2020, May 15). *Sunlight: Good For the Eyes as well as the Brain.* Dr. Phil Maffetone. *https://philmaffetone.com/sun-and-brain/*

Wikipedia contributors. (2024, June 12). *Biophilia hypothesis.* Wikipedia. *https://en.wikipedia.org/wiki/Biophilia_hypothesis*

Engemann, K., Pedersen, C. B., Arge, L., Tsirogiannis, C., Mortensen, P. B., & Svenning, J. (2019). Residential green space in childhood is associated with lower risk of psychiatric disorders from adolescence into adulthood. *Proceedings of the National Academy of Sciences of the United States of America, 116*(11), 5188–5193. *https://doi.org/10.1073/pnas.1807504116*

Barton, J., & Pretty, J. (2010). What is the Best Dose of Nature and Green Exercise for Improving Mental Health? A Multi-Study Analysis. *Environmental Science & Technology, 44*(10), 3947–3955. *https://doi.org/10.1021/es903183r*

Pasanen, T. P., Tyrväinen, L., & Korpela, K. M. (2014). The Relationship between Perceived Health and Physical Activity Indoors, Outdoors in Built Environments, and Outdoors in Nature. *Applied Psychology. Health and Well-being, 6*(3), 324–346. *https://doi.org/10.1111/aphw.12031*

Wikipedia contributors. (2024a, May 13). *Attention restoration theory.* Wikipedia. *https://en.wikipedia.org/wiki/Attention_restoration_theory#:~:text=Attention%20restoration%20theory%20claims%20that,stringent%20focus%20of%20everyday%20life*

The benefits of nature experience: Improved affect and cognition. (2015, March 3). The Nature and Health Alliance. *https://www.natureandhealthalliance.org/articles/2015/3/3/benefits-nature-experience-improved-affect-and-cognition*

Creating Community through Nature. (2022, June 7). American Camp Association. *https://www.acacamps.org/article/camping-magazine/creating-community-through-nature*

Dopko, R. L., Capaldi, C. A., & Zelenski, J. M. (2019). The psychological and social benefits of a nature experience for children: A preliminary investigation. *Journal of Environmental Psychology, 63,* 134–138. *https://doi.org/10.1016/j.jenvp.2019.05.002*

Experiencing God in Nature. (2019, April 3). Thomas Jay Oord. Retrieved July 9, 2024, from *https://thomasjayoord.com/index.php/blog/archives/experiencing-god-in-nature#_edn1*

The Cruise of the Corwin by John Muir. (n.d.). *https://vault.sierraclub.org/john_muir_exhibit/writings/cruise_of_the_corwin/chapter_4.aspx*

Whitworth, E. (2023, December 8). *Henry David Thoreau and Nature: Woods & wildlife at Walden Pond.* Shortform Books. *https://www.shortform.com/blog/henry-david-thoreau-and-nature/#:~:text=During%20his%20two%20years%20at,rhythms%20of%20the%20natural%20world*

Wright Brothers Impact: Biomimicry & the Birth of Aviation | Shapell. (2024, April 4). Shapell. *https://www.shapell.org/historical-perspectives/curated-manuscripts/the-wright-brothers-biomimicry-and-the-birth-of-aviation/*

Wikipedia contributors. (2024c, July 8). *Biomimetics.* Wikipedia. *https://en.wikipedia.org/wiki/Biomimetics#:~:text=Biomimetics%20or%20biomimicry%20is%20the,of%20solving%20complex%20human%20problems*

Mfa, R. J. S. (2020, September 18). *A hobby for all seasons: 7 Science-Backed Benefits of Indoor Plants.* Healthline. *https://www.healthline.com/health/healthy-home-guide/benefits-of-indoor-plants#7-benefits*

Yeo, N., White, M., Alcock, I., Garside, R., Dean, S., Smalley, A., &

Gatersleben, B. (2020). What is the best way of delivering virtual nature for improving mood? An experimental comparison of high definition TV, 360° video, and computer generated virtual reality. *Journal of Environmental Psychology, 72*, 101500. *https://doi.org/10.1016/j.jenvp.2020.101500*

Johnson, D. (n.d.). *"In every walk with nature one receives far more than he seeks" John Muir.* *https://blogs.georgefox.edu/dlgp/in-every-walk-with-nature-one-receives-far-more-than-he-seeks-john-muir/comment-page-1/*

Wood, H. (n.d.). *Quotations of John Muir – Writings – The John Muir Exhibit – Sierra Club. https://vault.sierraclub.org/john_muir_exhibit/writings/favorite_quotations.aspx#:~:text=In%20every%20walk%20with%20Nature,%2C%20John%2C%20%22Mormon%20Lilies.*